KETO DIET RECIPES

THE MOST DELICIOUS SELECTION OF SEAFOOD AND POULTRY RECIPES TO LOSE WEIGHT AND GET MORE ENERGY

JIMMY BOLTON

Table of Contents

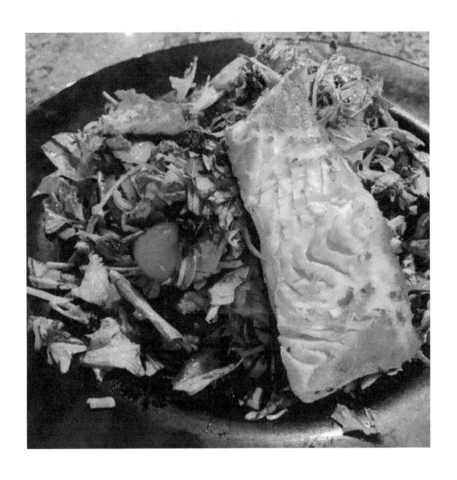

Introduction

Do you want to make a change in your life? Do you want to become a healthier person who can enjoy a new and improved life? Then, you are definitely in the right place. You are about to discover a wonderful and very healthy diet that has changed millions of lives. We are talking about the Ketogenic diet, a lifestyle that will mesmerize you and that will make you a new person in no time. So, let's sit back, relax and find out more about the Ketogenic diet.

A keto diet is a low carb one. This is the first and one of the most important things you should now. During such a diet, your body makes ketones in your liver and these are used as energy.
Your body will produce less insulin and glucose and a state of ketosis is induced.
Ketosis is a natural process that appears when our food intake is lower than usual. The body will soon adapt to this state and therefore you will be able to lose weight in no time but you will also become healthier and your physical and mental performances will improve.
Your blood sugar levels will improve and you won't be predisposed to diabetes.

Also, epilepsy and heart diseases can be prevented if you are on a Ketogenic diet.

Your cholesterol will improve and you will feel amazing in no time. How does that sound?

A Ketogenic diet is simple and easy to follow as long as you follow some simple rules. You don't need to make huge changes but there are some things you should know.

So, here goes!

If you are on a Ketogenic diet you can't eat:

- Grains like corn, cereals, rice, etc
- Fruits like bananas
- Sugar
- Dry beans
- Honey
- Potatoes
- Yams

If you are on a Ketogenic diet you can eat:

- Greens like spinach, green beans, kale, bok choy, etc
- Meat like poultry, fish, pork, lamb, beef, etc
- Eggs
- Above ground veggies like cauliflower or broccoli, napa cabbage or regular cabbage
- Nuts and seeds
- Cheese
- Ghee or butter
- Avocados and all kind of berries
- Sweeteners like erythritol, splenda, stevia and others that contain only a few carbs
- Coconut oil
- Avocado oil
- Olive oil

The list of foods you are allowed to eat during a keto diet is permissive and rich as you can see for yourself.

So, we think it should be pretty easy for you to start such a diet.

If you've made this choice already, then, it's time you checked our amazing keto recipe collection.

You will discover 50 of the best Ketogenic Seafood and Poultry recipes in the world and you will soon be able to make each and every one of these recipes.

Now let's start our magical culinary journey!
Ketogenic lifestyle...here we come!
Enjoy!

Seafood

Shrimp Stew

Have you ever tried something like this?

Preparation time: 10 minutes

Cooking time: 15 minutes

Servings: 6

Ingredients:

- ¼ cup yellow onion, chopped
- ¼ cup olive oil
- 1 garlic clove, minced
- 1 and ½ pounds shrimp, peeled and deveined
- ¼ cup red pepper, roasted and chopped
- 14 ounces canned tomatoes, chopped
- ¼ cup cilantro, chopped
- 2 tablespoons sriracha sauce
- 1 cup coconut milk
- Salt and black pepper to the taste
- 2 tablespoons lime juice

Directions:

1. Heat up a pan with the oil over medium heat, add onion, stir and cook for 4 minutes.

2. Add peppers and garlic, stir and cook for 4 minutes more.
3. Add cilantro, tomatoes and shrimp, stir and cook until shrimp turn pink.
4. Add coconut milk and sriracha sauce, stir and bring to a gentle simmer.
5. Add salt, pepper and lime juice, stir, transfer to bowls and serve.

Enjoy!

Nutrition: calories 250, fat 12, fiber 3, carbs 5, protein 20

Shrimp Alfredo

It looks unbelievable!

Preparation time: 10 minutes

Cooking time: 20 minutes

Servings: 4

Ingredients:

- 8 ounces mushrooms, chopped
- 1 asparagus bunch, cut into medium pieces
- 1 pound shrimp, peeled and deveined
- Salt and black pepper to the taste
- 1 spaghetti squash, cut in halves
- 2 tablespoons olive oil
- 2 teaspoons Italian seasoning
- 1 yellow onion, chopped
- 1 teaspoon red pepper flakes, crushed
- ¼ cup ghee
- 1 cup parmesan cheese, grated
- 2 garlic cloves, minced
- 1 cup heavy cream

Directions:

1. Place squash halves on a lined baking sheet, introduce in the oven at 425 degrees F and roast for 40 minutes.
2. Scoop insides and put into a bowl.
3. Put water in a pot, add some salt, bring to a boil over medium heat, add asparagus, steam for a couple of minutes, transfer to a bowl filled with ice water, drain and leave aside as well.
4. Heat up a pan with the oil over medium heat, add onions and mushrooms, stir and cook for 7 minutes.
5. Add pepper flakes, Italian seasoning, salt, pepper, squash and asparagus, stir and cook for a few minutes more.
6. Heat up another pan with the ghee over medium heat, add heavy cream, garlic and parmesan, stir and cook for 5 minutes.
7. Add shrimp to this pan, stir and cook for 7 minutes.
8. Divide veggies on plates, top with shrimp and sauce and serve.

Enjoy!

Nutrition: calories 455, fat 6, fiber 5, carbs 4, protein 13

Shrimp And Snow Peas Soup

It's one of the best ways to enjoy some shrimp!

Preparation time: 10 minutes

Cooking time: 10 minutes

Servings: 4

Ingredients:

- 4 scallions, chopped
- 1 and ½ tablespoons coconut oil
- 1 small ginger root, finely chopped
- 8 cups chicken stock
- ¼ cup coconut aminos
- 5 ounces canned bamboo shoots, sliced
- Black pepper to the taste
- ¼ teaspoon fish sauce
- 1 pound shrimp, peeled and deveined
- ½ pound snow peas
- 1 tablespoon sesame oil
- ½ tablespoon chili oil

Directions:

1. Heat up a pot with the coconut oil over medium heat, add scallions and ginger, stir and cook for 2 minutes.
2. Add coconut aminos, stock, black pepper and fish sauce, stir and bring to a boil.
3. Add shrimp, snow peas and bamboo shoots, stir and cook for 3 minutes.
4. Add sesame oil and hot chili oil, stir, divide into bowls and serve.

Enjoy!

Nutrition: calories 200, fat 3, fiber 2, carbs 4, protein 14

Simple Mussels Dish

You only need some simple ingredients to make a tasty and quick dish!

Preparation time: 5 minutes

Cooking time: 5 minutes

Servings: 4

Ingredients:

- 2 pound mussels, debearded and scrubbed
- 2 garlic cloves, minced
- 1 tablespoon ghee
- A splash of lemon juice

Directions:

1. Put some water in a pot, add mussels, bring to a boil over medium heat, cook for 5 minutes, take off heat, discard unopened mussels and transfer them to a bowl.
2. In another bowl, mix ghee with garlic and lemon juice, whisk and heat up in the microwave for 1 minute.
3. Pour over mussels and serve them right away.

Enjoy!

Nutrition: calories 50, fat 1, fiber 0, carbs 0.5, protein 2

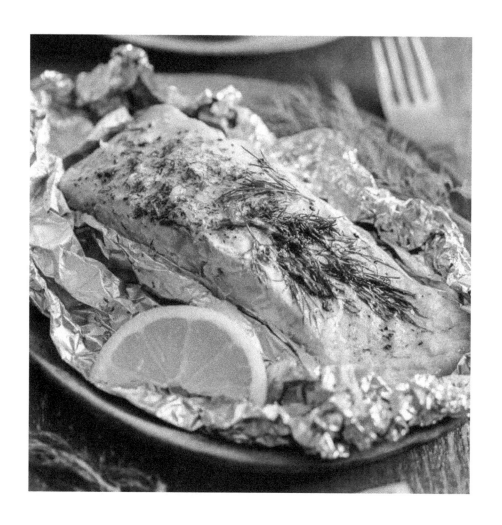

Simple Fried Calamari And Tasty Sauce

This is one of our favorite keto calamari dishes!

Preparation time: 10 minutes

Cooking time: 20 minutes

Servings: 2

Ingredients:

- 1 squid, cut into medium rings
- A pinch of cayenne pepper
- 1 egg, whisked
- 2 tablespoons coconut flour
- Salt and black pepper to the taste
- Coconut oil for frying
- 1 tablespoons lemon juice
- 4 tablespoons mayo
- 1 teaspoon sriracha sauce

Directions:

1. Season squid rings with salt, pepper and cayenne and put them in a bowl.
2. In a bowl, whisk the egg with salt, pepper and coconut flour and whisk well.

3. Dredge calamari rings in this mix.

4. Heat up a pan with enough coconut oil over medium heat, add calamari rings, cook them until they become gold on both sides.

5. Transfer to paper towels, drain grease and put in a bowl.

6. In another bowl, mix mayo with lemon juice and sriracha sauce, stir well and serve your calamari rings with this sauce on the side.

Enjoy!

Nutrition: calories 345, fat 32, fiber 3, carbs 3, protein 13

Baked Calamari And Shrimp

This Ketogenic seafood dish is great!

Preparation time: 10 minutes

Cooking time: 20 minutes

Servings: 1

Ingredients:

- 8 ounces calamari, cut into medium rings
- 7 ounces shrimp, peeled and deveined
- 1 eggs
- 3 tablespoons coconut flour
- 1 tablespoon coconut oil
- 2 tablespoons avocado, chopped
- 1 teaspoon tomato paste
- 1 tablespoon mayonnaise
- A splash of Worcestershire sauce
- 1 teaspoon lemon juice
- 2 lemon slices
- Salt and black pepper to the taste
- ½ teaspoon turmeric

Directions:

1. In a bowl, whisk the egg with coconut oil.
2. Add calamari rings and shrimp and toss to coat.
3. In another bowl, mix flour with salt, pepper and turmeric and stir.
4. Dredge calamari and shrimp in this mix, place everything on a lined baking sheet, introduce in the oven at 400 degrees F and bake for 10 minutes.
5. Flip calamari and shrimp and bake for 10 minutes more.
6. Meanwhile, in a bowl, mix avocado with mayo and tomato paste and mash using a fork.
7. Add Worcestershire sauce, lemon juice, salt and pepper and stir well.
8. Divide baked calamari and shrimp on plates and serve with the sauce and lemon juice on the side.

Enjoy!

Nutrition: calories 368, fat 23, fiber 3, carbs 10, protein 34

Octopus Salad

It's so fresh and light!

Preparation time: 10 minutes

Cooking time: 40 minutes

Servings: 2

Ingredients:

- 21 ounces octopus, rinsed
- Juice of 1 lemon
- 4 celery stalks, chopped
- 3 ounces olive oil
- Salt and black pepper to the taste
- 4 tablespoons parsley, chopped

Directions:

1. Put the octopus in a pot, add water to cover, cover pot, bring to a boil over medium heat, cook for 40 minutes, drain and leave aside to cool down.
2. Chop octopus and put it in a salad bowl.
3. Add celery stalks, parsley, oil and lemon juice and toss well.
4. Season with salt and pepper, toss again and serve.

Enjoy!

Nutrition: calories 140, fat 10, fiber 3, carbs 6, protein 23

Clam Chowder

It's perfect for a very cold winter day!

Preparation time: 10 minutes

Cooking time: 2 hours

Servings: 4

Ingredients:

- 1 cup celery stalks, chopped
- Salt and black pepper to the taste
- 1 teaspoon thyme, ground
- 2 cups chicken stock
- 14 ounces canned baby clams
- 2 cups whipping cream
- 1 cup onion, chopped
- 13 bacon slices, chopped

Directions:

1. Heat up a pan over medium heat, add bacon slices, brown them and transfer to a bowl.
2. Heat up the same pan over medium heat, add celery and onion, stir and cook for 5 minutes.

3. Transfer everything to your Crockpot, also add bacon, baby clams, salt, pepper, stock, thyme and whipping cream, stir and cook on High for 2 hours.

4. Divide into bowls and serve.

Enjoy!

Nutrition: calories 420, fat 22, fiber 0, carbs 5, protein 25

Delicious Flounder And Shrimp

You just got the opportunity to learn an amazing keto recipe!

Preparation time: 10 minutes

Cooking time: 20 minutes

Servings: 4

Ingredients:

For the seasoning:

- 2 teaspoons onion powder
- 2 teaspoons thyme, dried
- 2 teaspoons sweet paprika
- 2 teaspoons garlic powder
- Salt and black pepper to the taste
- ½ teaspoon allspice, ground
- 1 teaspoon oregano, dried
- A pinch of cayenne pepper
- ¼ teaspoon nutmeg, ground
- ¼ teaspoon cloves
- A pinch of cinnamon powder

For the etouffee:

- 2 shallots, chopped
- 1 tablespoon ghee
- 8 ounces bacon, sliced
- 1 green bell pepper, chopped
- 1 celery stick, chopped
- 2 tablespoons coconut flour
- 1 tomato, chopped
- 4 garlic cloves, minced
- 8 ounces shrimp, peeled, deveined and chopped
- 2 cups chicken stock
- 1 tablespoon coconut milk
- A handful parsley, chopped
- 1 teaspoon Tabasco sauce
- Salt and black pepper to the taste

For the flounder:

- 4 flounder fillets
- 2 tablespoons ghee

Directions:

1. In a bowl, mix paprika with thyme, garlic and onion powder, salt, pepper, oregano, allspice, cayenne pepper, cloves, nutmeg and cinnamon and stir.
2. Reserve 2 tablespoons of this mix, rub the flounder with the rest and leave aside.
3. Heat up a pan over medium heat, add bacon, stir and cook for 6 minutes.
4. Add celery, bell pepper, shallots and 1 tablespoon ghee, stir and cook for 4 minutes.
5. Add tomato and garlic, stir and cook for 4 minutes.
6. Add coconut flour and reserved seasoning, stir and cook for 2 minutes more.
7. Add chicken stock and bring to a simmer.
8. Meanwhile, heat up a pan with 2 tablespoons ghee over medium high heat, add fish, cook for 2 minutes, flip and cut for 2 minutes more.

9. Add shrimp to the pan with the stock, stir and cook for 2 minutes.
10. Add parsley, salt, pepper, coconut milk and Tabasco sauce, stir and take off heat.
11. Divide fish on plates, top with the shrimp sauce and serve.

Enjoy!

Nutrition: calories 200, fat 5, fiber 7, carbs 4, protein 20

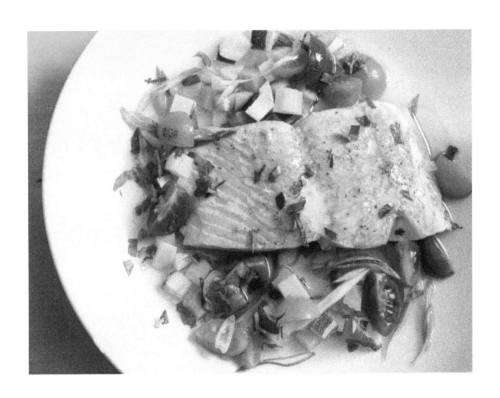

Shrimp Salad

Serve this fresh salad tonight for dinner!

Preparation time: 10 minutes

Cooking time: 10 minutes

Servings: 4

Ingredients:

- 2 tablespoons olive oil
- 1 pound shrimp, peeled and deveined
- Salt and black pepper to the taste
- 2 tablespoons lime juice
- 3 endives, leaves separated
- 3 tablespoons parsley, chopped
- 2 teaspoons mint, chopped
- 1 tablespoon tarragon, chopped
- 1 tablespoon lemon juice
- 2 tablespoons mayonnaise
- 1 teaspoon lime zest
- ½ cup sour cream

Directions:

1. In a bowl, mix shrimp with salt, pepper and the olive oil, toss to coat and spread them on a lined baking sheet.
2. Introduce shrimp in the oven at 400 degrees F and bake for 10 minutes.
3. Add lime juice, toss them to coat again and leave aside for now.
4. In a bowl, mix mayo with sour cream, lime zest, lemon juice, salt, pepper, tarragon, mint and parsley and stir very well.
5. Chop shrimp, add to salad dressing, toss to coat everything and spoon into endive leaves.
6. Serve right away.

Enjoy!

Nutrition: calories 200, fat 11, fiber 2, carbs 1, protein 13

Delicious Oysters

This special and flavored dish is here to impress you!

Preparation time: 10 minutes

Cooking time: 0 minutes

Servings: 4

Ingredients:

- 12 oysters, shucked
- Juice of 1 lemon
- Juice from 1 orange
- Zest from 1 orange
- Juice from 1 lime
- Zest from 1 lime
- 2 tablespoons ketchup
- 1 Serrano chili pepper, chopped
- 1 cup tomato juice
- ½ teaspoon ginger, grated
- ¼ teaspoon garlic, minced
- Salt to the taste
- ¼ cup olive oil
- ¼ cup cilantro, chopped

- ¼ cup scallions, chopped

Directions:

1. In a bowl, mix lemon juice, orange juice, orange zest, lime juice and zest, ketchup, chili pepper, tomato juice, ginger, garlic, oil, scallions, cilantro and salt and stir well.
2. Spoon this into oysters and serve them.

Enjoy!

Nutrition: calories 100, fat 1, fiber 0, carbs 2, protein 5

Incredible Salmon Rolls

This Asian dish is just delicious!

Preparation time: 10 minutes

Cooking time: 0 minutes

Servings: 12

Ingredients:

- 2 nori seeds
- 1 small avocado, pitted, peeled and finely chopped
- 6 ounces smoked salmon. Sliced
- 4 ounces cream cheese
- 1 cucumber, sliced
- 1 teaspoon wasabi paste
- Picked ginger for serving

Directions:

1. Place nori sheets on a sushi mat.
2. Divide salmon slices on them and also avocado and cucumber slices.
3. In a bowl, mix cream cheese with wasabi paste and stir well.

4. Spread this over cucumber slices, roll your nori sheets, press well, cut each into 6 pieces and serve with pickled ginger.

Enjoy!

Nutrition: calories 80, fat 6, fiber 1, carbs 2, protein 4

Salmon Skewers

These are easy to make and they are very healthy!

Preparation time: 10 minutes

Cooking time: 8 minutes

Servings: 4

Ingredients:

- 12 ounces salmon fillet, cubed
- 1 red onion, cut into chunks
- ½ red bell pepper cut in chunks
- ½ green bell pepper cut in chunks
- ½ orange bell pepper cut in chunks
- Juice from 1 lemon
- Salt and black pepper to the taste
- A drizzle of olive oil

Directions:

1. Thread skewers with onion, red, green and orange pepper and salmon cubes.
2. Season them with salt and pepper, drizzle oil and lemon juice and place them on preheated grill over medium high heat.

3. Cook for 4 minutes on each side, divide between plates and serve.

Enjoy!

Nutrition: calories 150, fat 3, fiber 6, carbs 3, protein 8

Grilled Shrimp

This is perfect! Just check it out!

Preparation time: 20 minutes

Cooking time: 10 minutes

Servings: 4

Ingredients:

- 1 pound shrimp, peeled and deveined
- 1 tablespoon lemon juice
- 1 garlic clove, minced
- ½ cup basil leaves
- 1 tablespoon pine nuts, toasted
- 2 tablespoons parmesan, grated
- 2 tablespoons olive oil
- Salt and black pepper to the taste

Directions:

1. In your food processor, mix parmesan with basil, garlic, pine nuts, oil, salt, pepper and lemon juice and blend well.
2. Transfer this to a bowl, add shrimp, toss to coat and leave aside for 20 minutes.

3. Thread skewers with marinated shrimp, place them on preheated grill over medium high heat, cook for 3 minutes, flip and cook for 3 more minutes.
4. Arrange on plates and serve.

Enjoy!

Nutrition: calories 185, fat 11, fiber 0, carbs 2, protein 13

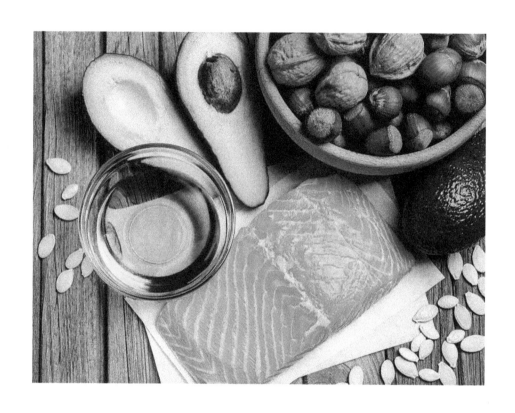

Calamari Salad

It's an excellent choice for a summer day!

Preparation time: 30 minutes

Cooking time: 4 minutes

Servings: 4

Ingredients:

- 2 long red chilies, chopped
- 2 small red chilies, chopped
- 2 garlic cloves, minced
- 3 green onions, chopped
- 1 tablespoon balsamic vinegar
- Salt and black pepper to the taste
- Juice of 1 lemon
- 6 pounds calamari hoods, tentacles reserved
- 3.5 ounces olive oil
- 3 ounces rocket for serving

Directions:

1. In a bowl, mix long red chilies with small red chilies, green onions, vinegar, half of the oil, garlic, salt, pepper and lemon juice and stir well.

45

2. Place calamari and tentacles in a bowl, season with salt and pepper, drizzle the rest of the oil, toss to coat and place on preheated grill over medium high heat.
3. Cook for 2 minutes on each side and transfer to the chili marinade you've made.
4. Toss to coat and leave aside for 30 minutes.
5. Arrange rocket on plates, top with calamari and its marinade and serve.

Enjoy!

Nutrition: calories 200, fat 4, fiber 2, carbs 2, protein 7

Cod Salad

It's always worth trying something new!

Preparation time: 2 hours and 10 minutes

Cooking time: 20 minutes

Servings: 8

Ingredients:

- 2 cups jarred pimiento peppers, chopped
- 2 pounds salt cod
- 1 cup parsley, chopped
- 1 cup kalamata olives, pitted and chopped
- 6 tablespoons capers
- ¾ cup olive oil
- Salt and black pepper to the taste
- Juice from 2 lemons
- 4 garlic cloves, minced
- 2 celery ribs, chopped
- ½ teaspoon red chili flakes
- 1 escarole head, leaves separated

Directions:

1. Put cod in a pot, add water to cover, bring to a boil over medium heat, boil for 20 minutes, drain and cut into medium chunks.
2. Put cod in a salad bowl, add peppers, parsley, olives, capers, celery, garlic, lemon juice, salt, pepper, olive oil and chili flakes and toss to coat.
3. Arrange escarole leaves on a platter, add cod salad and serve.

Enjoy!

Nutrition: calories 240, fat 4, fiber 2, carbs 6, protein 9

Sardines Salad

It's a rich and nutritious winter salad you have to try soon!

Preparation time: 10 minutes

Cooking time: 0 minutes

Servings: 1

Ingredients:

- 5 ounces canned sardines in oil
- 1 tablespoons lemon juice
- 1 small cucumber, chopped
- ½ tablespoon mustard
- Salt and black pepper to the taste

Directions:

1. Drain sardines, put them in a bowl and mash using a fork.
2. Add salt, pepper, cucumber, lemon juice and mustard, stir well and serve cold.

Enjoy!

Nutrition: calories 200, fat 20, fiber 1, carbs 0, protein 20

Italian Clams Delight

It's a special Italian delight! Serve this amazing dish to your family!

Preparation time: 10 minutes

Cooking time: 10 minutes

Servings: 6

Ingredients:

- ½ cup ghee
- 36 clams, scrubbed
- 1 teaspoon red pepper flakes, crushed
- 1 teaspoon parsley, chopped
- 5 garlic cloves, minced
- 1 tablespoon oregano, dried
- 2 cups white wine

Directions:

1. Heat up a pan with the ghee over medium heat, add garlic, stir and cook for 1 minute.
2. Add parsley, oregano, wine and pepper flakes and stir well.
3. Add clams, stir, cover and cook for 10 minutes.

4. Discard unopened clams, ladle clams and their mix into bowls and serve.

Enjoy!

Nutrition: calories 224, fat 15, fiber 2, carbs 3, protein 4

Orange Glazed Salmon

You must try this soon! It's a delicious keto fish recipe!

Preparation time: 10 minutes

Cooking time: 10 minutes

Servings: 2

Ingredients:

- 2 lemons, sliced
- 1 pound wild salmon, skinless and cubed
- ¼ cup balsamic vinegar
- ¼ cup red orange juice
- 1 teaspoon coconut oil
- 1/3 cup orange marmalade, no sugar added

Directions:

1. Heat up a pot over medium heat, add vinegar, orange juice and marmalade, stir well, bring to a simmer for 1 minute, reduce temperature, cook until it thickens a bit and take off heat.
2. Arrange salmon and lemon slices on skewers and brush them on one side with the orange glaze.

3. Brush your kitchen grill with coconut oil and heat up over medium heat.
4. Place salmon kebabs on grill with glazed side down and cook for 4 minutes.
5. Flip kebabs, brush them with the rest of the orange glaze and cook for 4 minutes more.
6. Serve right away.

Enjoy!

Nutrition: calories 160, fat 3, fiber 2, carbs 1, protein 8

Delicious Tuna And Chimichurri Sauce

Who wouldn't love this keto dish?

Preparation time: 10 minutes

Cooking time: 5 minutes

Servings: 4

Ingredients:

- ½ cup cilantro, chopped
- 1/3 cup olive oil
- 2 tablespoons olive oil
- 1 small red onion, chopped
- 3 tablespoon balsamic vinegar
- 2 tablespoons parsley, chopped
- 2 tablespoons basil, chopped
- 1 jalapeno pepper, chopped
- 1 pound sushi grade tuna steak
- Salt and black pepper to the taste
- 1 teaspoon red pepper flakes
- 1 teaspoon thyme, chopped
- A pinch of cayenne pepper
- 3 garlic cloves, minced

- 2 avocados, pitted, peeled and sliced
- 6 ounces baby arugula

Directions:

1. In a bowl, mix 1/3 cup oil with jalapeno, vinegar, onion, cilantro, basil, garlic, parsley, pepper flakes, thyme, cayenne, salt and pepper, whisk well and leave aside for now.
2. Heat up a pan with the rest of the oil over medium high heat, add tuna, season with salt and pepper, cook for 2 minutes on each side, transfer to a cutting board, leave aside to cool down a bit and slice.
3. Mix arugula with half of the chimichurri mix you've made and toss to coat.
4. Divide arugula on plates, top with tuna slices, drizzle the rest of the chimichurri sauce and serve with avocado slices on the side.

Enjoy!

Nutrition: calories 186, fat 3, fiber 1, carbs 4, protein 20

Salmon Bites And Chili Sauce

This is an amazing and super tasty combination!

Preparation time: 10 minutes

Cooking time: 15 minutes

Servings: 6

Ingredients:

- 1 and ¼ cups coconut, desiccated and unsweetened
- 1 pound salmon, cubed
- 1 egg
- Salt and black pepper
- 1 tablespoon water
- 1/3 cup coconut flour
- 3 tablespoons coconut oil

For the sauce:

- ¼ teaspoon agar agar
- 3 garlic cloves, chopped
- ¾ cup water
- 4 Thai red chilies, chopped
- ¼ cup balsamic vinegar
- ½ cup stevia

- A pinch of salt

Directions:

1. In a bowl, mix flour with salt and pepper and stir.
2. In another bowl, whisk egg and 1 tablespoon water.
3. Put the coconut in a third bowl.
4. Dip salmon cubes in flour, egg and then in coconut and place them on a plate.
5. Heat up a pan with the coconut oil over medium high heat, add salmon bites, cook for 3 minutes on each side and transfer them to paper towels.
6. Heat up a pan with ¾ cup water over high heat, sprinkle agar agar and bring to a boil.
7. Cook for 3 minutes and take off heat.
8. In your blender, mix garlic with chilies, vinegar, stevia and a pinch of salt and blend well.
9. Transfer this to a small pan and heat up over medium high heat.
10. Stir, add agar mix and cook for 3 minutes.
11. Serve your salmon bites with chili sauce on the side.

Enjoy!

Nutrition: calories 50, fat 2, fiber 0, carbs 4, protein 2

Irish Clams

It's an excellent idea for your dinner!

Preparation time: 10 minutes

Cooking time: 10 minutes

Servings: 4

Ingredients:

- 2 pounds clams, scrubbed
- 3 ounces pancetta
- 1 tablespoon olive oil
- 3 tablespoons ghee
- 2 garlic cloves, minced
- 1 bottle infused cider
- Salt and black pepper to the taste
- Juice of ½ lemon
- 1 small green apple, chopped
- 2 thyme springs, chopped

Directions:

1. Heat up a pan with the oil over medium high heat, add pancetta, brown for 3 minutes and reduce temperature to medium.

2. Add ghee, garlic, salt, pepper and shallot, stir and cook for 3 minutes.

3. Increase heat again, add cider, stir well and cook for 1 minute.

4. Add clams and thyme, cover pan and simmer for 5 minutes.

5. Discard unopened clams, add lemon juice and apple pieces, stir and divide into bowls.

6. Serve hot.

Enjoy!

Nutrition: calories 100, fat 2, fiber 1, carbs 1, protein 20

Seared Scallops And Roasted Grapes

A special occasion requires a special dish! Try these keto scallops!

Preparation time: 5 minutes

Cooking time: 10 minutes

Servings: 4

Ingredients:

- 1 pound scallops
- 3 tablespoons olive oil
- 1 shallot, chopped
- 3 garlic cloves, minced
- 2 cups spinach
- 1 cup chicken stock
- 1 romanesco lettuce head
- 1 and ½ cups red grapes, cut in halves
- ¼ cup walnuts, toasted and chopped
- 1 tablespoon ghee
- Salt and black pepper to the taste

Directions:

1. Put romanesco in your food processor, blend and transfer to a bowl.

2. Heat up a pan with 2 tablespoons oil over medium high heat, add shallot and garlic, stir and cook for 1 minute.
3. Add romanesco, spinach and 1 cup stock, stir, cook for 3 minutes, blend using an immersion blender and take off heat.
4. Heat up another pan with 1 tablespoon oil and the ghee over medium high heat, add scallops, season with salt and pepper, cook for 2 minutes, flip and sear for 1 minute more.
5. Divide romanesco mix on plates, add scallops on the side, top with walnuts and grapes and serve.

Enjoy!

Nutrition: calories 300, fat 12, fiber 2, carbs 6, protein 20

Oysters And Pico De Gallo

It's flavored and very delicious!

Preparation time: 10 minutes

Cooking time: 10 minutes

Servings: 6

Ingredients:

- 18 oysters, scrubbed
- A handful cilantro, chopped
- 2 tomatoes, chopped
- 1 jalapeno pepper, chopped
- ¼ cup red onion, finely chopped
- Salt and black pepper to the taste
- ½ cup Monterey Jack cheese, shredded
- 2 limes, cut into wedges
- Juice from 1 lime

Directions:

1. In a bowl, mix onion with jalapeno, cilantro, tomatoes, salt, pepper and lime juice and stir well.
2. Place oysters on preheated grill over medium high heat, cover grill and cook for 7 minutes until they open.

3. Transfer opened oysters to a heatproof dish and discard unopened ones.

4. Top oysters with cheese and introduce in preheated broiler for 1 minute.

5. Arrange oysters on a platter, top each with tomatoes mix you've made earlier and serve with lime wedges on the side.

Enjoy!

Nutrition: calories 70, fat 2, fiber 0, carbs 1, protein 1

Grilled Squid And Tasty Guacamole

The squid combines perfectly with the delicious guacamole!

Preparation time: 10 minutes

Cooking time: 10 minutes

Servings: 2

Ingredients:

- 2 medium squids, tentacles separated and tubes scored lengthwise
- A drizzle of olive oil
- Juice from 1 lime
- Salt and black pepper to the taste

For the guacamole:

- 2 avocados, pitted, peeled and chopped
- Some coriander springs, chopped
- 2 red chilies, chopped
- 1 tomato, chopped
- 1 red onion, chopped
- Juice from 2 limes

Directions:

1. Season squid and squid tentacles with salt, pepper, drizzle some olive oil and massage well.
2. Place on preheated grill over medium high heat score side down and cook for 2 minutes.
3. Flip and cook for 2 minutes more and transfer to a bowl.
4. Add juice from 1 lime, toss to coat and keep warm.
5. Put avocado in a bowl and mash using a fork.
6. Add coriander, chilies, tomato, onion and juice from 2 limes and stir well everything.
7. Divide squid on plates, top with guacamole and serve.

Enjoy!

Nutrition: calories 500, fat 43, fiber 6, carbs 7, protein 20

Shrimp And Cauliflower Delight

It looks good and it tastes amazing!

Preparation time: 10 minutes

Cooking time: 15 minutes

Servings: 2

Ingredients:

- 1 tablespoon ghee
- 1 cauliflower head, florets separated
- 1 pound shrimp, peeled and deveined
- ¼ cup coconut milk
- 8 ounces mushrooms, roughly chopped
- A pinch of red pepper flakes
- Salt and black pepper to the taste
- 2 garlic cloves, minced
- 4 bacon slices
- ½ cup beef stock
- 1 tablespoon parsley, finely chopped
- 1 tablespoon chives, chopped

Directions:

1. Heat up a pan over medium high heat, add bacon, cook until it's crispy, transfer to paper towels and leave aside.
2. Heat up another pan with 1 tablespoon bacon fat over medium high heat, add shrimp, cook for 2 minutes on each side and transfer to a bowl.
3. Heat up the pan again over medium heat, add mushrooms, stir and cook for 3-4 minutes.
4. Add garlic, pepper flakes, stir and cook for 1 minute.
5. Add beef stock, salt, pepper and return shrimp to pan as well.
6. Stir, cook until everything thickens a bit, take off heat and keep warm.
7. Meanwhile, put cauliflower in your food processor and mince it.
8. Place this into a heated pan over medium high heat, stir and cook for 5 minutes.
9. Add ghee and butter, stir and blend using an immersion blender.
10. Add salt and pepper to the taste, stir and divide into bowls.
11. Top with shrimp mix and serve with parsley and chives sprinkled all over.

Enjoy!

Nutrition: calories 245, fat 7, fiber 4, carbs 6, protein 20

Salmon Stuffed With Shrimp

It will soon become one of your favorite keto recipes!

Preparation time: 10 minutes

Cooking time: 25 minutes

Servings: 2

Ingredients:

- 2 salmon fillets
- A drizzle of olive oil
- 5 ounces tiger shrimp, peeled, deveined and chopped
- 6 mushrooms, chopped
- 3 green onions, chopped
- 2 cups spinach
- ¼ cup macadamia nuts, toasted and chopped
- Salt and black pepper to the taste
- A pinch of nutmeg
- ¼ cup mayonnaise

Directions:

1. Heat up a pan with the oil over medium high heat, add mushrooms, onions, salt and pepper, stir and cook for 4 minutes.

2. Add macadamia nuts, stir and cook for 2 minutes.

3. Add spinach, stir and cook for 1 minute.

4. Add shrimp, stir and cook for 1 minutes.

5. Take off heat, leave aside for a few minutes, add mayo and nutmeg and stir well.

6. Make an incision lengthwise in each salmon fillet, sprinkle salt and pepper, divide spinach and shrimp mix into incisions and place on a working surface.

7. Heat up a pan with a drizzle of oil over medium high heat, add stuffed salmon, skin side down, cook for 1 minutes, reduce temperature, cover pan and cook for 8 minutes.

8. Broil for 3 minutes, divide between plates and serve.

Enjoy!

Nutrition: calories 430, fat 30, fiber 3, carbs 7, protein 50

Mustard Glazed Salmon

This is one of our favorite keto salmon dishes! You will feel the same!

Preparation time: 10 minutes

Cooking time: 20 minutes

Servings: 1

Ingredients:

- 1 big salmon fillet
- Salt and black pepper to the taste
- 2 tablespoons mustard
- 1 tablespoon coconut oil
- 1 tablespoon maple extract

Directions:

1. In a bowl, mix maple extract with mustard and whisk well.
2. Season salmon with salt and pepper and brush salmon with half of the mustard mix
3. Heat up a pan with the oil over medium high heat, place salmon flesh side down and cook for 5 minutes.

4. Brush salmon with the rest of the mustard mix, transfer to a baking dish, introduce in the oven at 425 degrees F and bake for 15 minutes.
5. Serve with a tasty side salad.

Enjoy!

Nutrition: calories 240, fat 7, fiber 1, carbs 5, protein 23

Incredible Salmon Dish

You will make this over and over again!

Preparation time: 10 minutes

Cooking time: 15 minutes

Servings: 4

Ingredients:

- 3 cups ice water
- 2 teaspoons sriracha sauce
- 4 teaspoons stevia
- 3 scallions, chopped
- Salt and black pepper to the taste
- 2 teaspoons flaxseed oil
- 4 teaspoons apple cider vinegar
- 3 teaspoons avocado oil
- 4 medium salmon fillets
- 4 cups baby arugula
- 2 cups cabbage, finely chopped
- 1 and ½ teaspoon Jamaican jerk seasoning
- ¼ cup pepitas, toasted
- 2 cups watermelon radish, julienned

Directions:

1. Put ice water in a bowl, add scallions and leave aside.
2. In another bowl, mix sriracha sauce with stevia and stir well.
3. Transfer 2 teaspoons of this mix to a bowl and mix with half of the avocado oil, flaxseed oil, vinegar, salt and pepper and whisk well.
4. Sprinkle jerk seasoning over salmon, rub with sriracha and stevia mix and season with salt and pepper.
5. Heat up a pan with the rest of the avocado oil over medium high heat, add salmon, flesh side down, cook for 4 minutes, flip and cook for 4 minutes more and divide between plates.
6. In a bowl, mix radishes with cabbage and arugula.
7. Add salt, pepper, sriracha and vinegar mix and toss well.
8. Add this next to salmon fillets, drizzle the remaining sriracha and stevia sauce all over and top with pepitas and drained scallions.

Enjoy!

Nutrition: calories 160, fat 6, fiber 1, carbs 1, protein 12

Scallops And Fennel Sauce

It contains a lot of healthy elements and it's easy to make! Try it if you are on a keto diet!

Preparation time: 10 minutes

Cooking time: 10 minutes

Servings: 2

Ingredients:

- 6 scallops
- 1 fennel, trimmed, leaves chopped and bulbs cut into wedges
- Juice of ½ lime
- 1 lime, cut into wedges
- Zest from 1 lime
- 1 egg yolk
- 3 tablespoons ghee, melted and heated up
- ½ tablespoons olive oil
- Salt and black pepper to the taste

Directions:

1. Season scallops with salt and pepper, put in a bowl and mix with half of the lime juice and half of the zest and toss to coat.
2. In a bowl, mix egg yolk with some salt and pepper, the rest of the lime juice and the rest of the lime zest and whisk well.
3. Add melted ghee and stir very well.
4. Also add fennel leaves and stir.
5. Brush fennel wedges with oil, place on heated grill over medium high heat, cook for 2 minutes, flip and cook for 2 minutes more.
6. Add scallops on the grill, cook for 2 minutes, flip and cook for 2 minutes more.
7. Divide fennel and scallops on plates, drizzle fennel and ghee mix and serve with lime wedges on the side.

Enjoy!

Nutrition: calories 400, fat 24, fiber 4, carbs 12, protein 25

Salmon And Lemon Relish

Enjoy a slow cooked salmon and a delicious relish!

Preparation time: 10 minutes

Cooking time: 1 hour

Servings: 2

Ingredients:

- 2 medium salmon fillets
- Salt and black pepper to the taste
- A drizzle of olive oil
- 1 shallot, chopped
- 1 tablespoon lemon juice
- 1 big lemon
- ¼ cup olive oil
- 2 tablespoons parsley, finely chopped

Directions:

1. Brush salmon fillets with a drizzle of olive oil, sprinkle with salt and pepper, place on a lined baking sheet, introduce in the oven at 400 degrees F and bake for 1 hour.

2. Meanwhile, put shallot in a bowl, add 1 tablespoon lemon juice, salt and pepper, stir and leave aside for 10 minutes.
3. Cut the whole lemon into wedges and then very thinly.
4. Add this to shallots, also add parsley and ¼ cup olive oil and stir everything.
5. Take salmon out of the oven, break into medium pieces and serve with the lemon relish on the side.

Enjoy!

Nutrition: calories 200, fat 10, fiber 1, carbs 5, protein 20

Mussels Soup

Oh my God! This is so good!

Preparation time: 10 minutes

Cooking time: 15 minutes

Servings: 6

Ingredients:

- 2 pounds mussels
- 28 ounces canned tomatoes, crushed
- 28 ounces canned tomatoes, chopped
- 2 cup chicken stock
- 1 teaspoon red pepper flakes, crushed
- 3 garlic cloves, minced
- 1 handful parsley, chopped
- 1 yellow onion, chopped
- Salt and black pepper to the taste
- 1 tablespoon olive oil

Directions:

1. Heat up a Dutch oven with the oil over medium high heat, add onion, stir and cook for 3 minutes.

2. Add garlic and red pepper flakes, stir and cook for 1 minute.
3. Add crushed and chopped tomatoes and stir.
4. Add chicken stock, salt and pepper, stir and bring to a boil.
5. Add rinsed mussels, salt and pepper, cook until they open, discard unopened ones and mix with parsley.
6. Stir, divide into bowls and serve.

Enjoy!

Nutrition: calories 250, fat 3, fiber 3, carbs 2, protein 8

Swordfish And Mango Salsa

The mango salsa is divine! Just serve it with the swordfish!

Preparation time: 10 minutes

Cooking time: 6 minutes

Servings: 2

Ingredients:

- 2 medium swordfish steaks
- Salt and black pepper to the taste
- 2 teaspoons avocado oil
- 1 tablespoon cilantro, chopped
- 1 mango, chopped
- 1 avocado, pitted, peeled and chopped
- A pinch of cumin
- A pinch of onion powder
- A pinch of garlic powder
- 1 orange, peeled and sliced
- ½ balsamic vinegar

Directions:

1. Season fish steaks with salt, pepper, garlic powder, onion powder and cumin.

2. Heat up a pan with half of the oil over medium high heat, add fish steaks and cook them for 3 minutes on each side.
3. Meanwhile, in a bowl, mix avocado with mango, cilantro, balsamic vinegar, salt, pepper and the rest of the oil and stir well.
4. Divide fish on plates, top with mango salsa and serve with orange slices on the side.

Enjoy!

Nutrition: calories 160, fat 3, fiber 2, carbs 4, protein 8

Tasty Sushi Bowl

It's a tasty recipe full of great ingredients!

Preparation time: 10 minutes

Cooking time: 7 minutes

Servings: 4

Ingredients:

- 1 ahi tuna steak
- 2 tablespoons coconut oil
- 1 cauliflower head, florets separated
- 2 tablespoons green onions, chopped
- 1 avocado, pitted, peeled and chopped
- 1 cucumber, grated
- 1 nori sheet, torn
- Some cloves sprouts

For the salad dressing:

- 1 tablespoon sesame oil
- 2 tablespoons coconut aminos
- 1 tablespoon apple cider vinegar
- A pinch of salt
- 1 teaspoon stevia

Directions:

1. Put cauliflower florets in your food processor and blend until you obtain a cauliflower "rice".
2. Put some water in a pot, add a steamer basket inside, add cauliflower rice, bring to a boil over medium heat, cover, steam for a few minutes, drain and transfer "rice" to a bowl.
3. Heat up a pan with the coconut oil over medium high heat, add tuna, cook for 1 minute on each side and transfer to a cutting board.
4. Divide cauliflower rice into bowls, top with nori pieces, cloves sprouts, cucumber, green onions and avocado.
5. In a bowl, mix sesame oil with vinegar, coconut aminos, salt and stevia and whisk well.
6. Drizzle this over cauliflower rice and mixed veggies, top with tuna pieces and serve.

Enjoy!

Nutrition: calories 300, fat 12, fiber 6, carbs 6, protein 15

Tasty Grilled Swordfish

You don't need to be an expert cook to make this tasty keto dish!

Preparation time: 3 hours and 10 minutes

Cooking time: 10 minutes

Servings: 4

Ingredients:

- 1 tablespoon parsley, chopped
- 1 lemon, cut into wedges
- 4 swordfish steaks
- 3 garlic cloves, minced
- 1/3 cup chicken stock
- 3 tablespoons olive oil
- ¼ cup lemon juice
- Salt and black pepper to the taste
- ½ teaspoon rosemary, dried
- ½ teaspoon sage, dried
- ½ teaspoon marjoram, dried

Directions:

1. In a bowl, mix chicken stock with garlic, lemon juice, olive oil, salt, pepper, sage, marjoram and rosemary and whisk well.

2. Add swordfish steaks, toss to coat and keep in the fridge for 3 hours.
3. Place marinated fish steaks on preheated grill over medium high heat and cook for 5 minutes on each side.
4. Arrange on plates, sprinkle parsley on to and serve with lemon wedges on the side.

Enjoy!

Nutrition: calories 136, fat 5, fiber 0, carbs 1, protein 20

Ketogenic Poultry Recipes

Delicious Chicken Nuggets

This is perfect for a friendly meal!

Preparation time: 10 minutes

Cooking time: 15 minutes

Servings: 2

Ingredients:

- ½ cup coconut flour
- 1 egg
- 2 tablespoons garlic powder
- 2 chicken breasts, cubed
- Salt and black pepper to the taste
- ½ cup ghee

Directions:

1. In a bowl, mix garlic powder with coconut flour, salt and pepper and stir.
2. In another bowl, whisk egg well.
3. Dip chicken breast cubes in egg mix, then in flour mix.
4. Heat up a pan with the ghee over medium heat, drop chicken nuggets and cook them for 5 minutes on each side.

5. Transfer to paper towels, drain grease and then serve them with some tasty ketchup on the side.

Enjoy!

Nutrition: calories 60, fat 3, fiber 0.2, carbs 3, protein 4

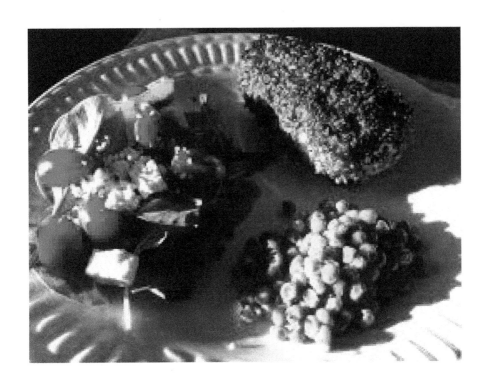

Chicken Wings And Tasty Mint Chutney

It's so fresh and delicious!

Preparation time: 20 minutes

Cooking time: 25 minutes

Servings: 6

Ingredients:

- 18 chicken wings, cut in halves
- 1 tablespoon turmeric
- 1 tablespoon cumin, ground
- 1 tablespoon ginger, grated
- 1 tablespoon coriander, ground
- 1 tablespoon paprika
- A pinch of cayenne pepper
- Salt and black pepper to the taste
- 2 tablespoons olive oil

For the chutney:

- Juice of ½ lime
- 1 cup mint leaves
- 1 small ginger piece, chopped
- ¾ cup cilantro

- 1 tablespoon olive oil
- 1 tablespoon water
- Salt and black pepper to the taste
- 1 Serrano pepper

Directions:

1. In a bowl, mix 1 tablespoon ginger with cumin, coriander, paprika, turmeric, salt, pepper, cayenne and 2 tablespoons oil and stir well.
2. Add chicken wings pieces to this mix, toss to coat well and keep in the fridge for 20 minutes.
3. Heat up your grill over high heat, add marinated wings, cook for 25 minutes, turning them from time to time and transfer to a bowl.
4. In your blender, mix mint with cilantro, 1 small ginger pieces, juice from ½ lime, 1 tablespoon olive oil, salt, pepper, water and Serrano pepper and blend very well.
5. Serve your chicken wings with this sauce on the side.

Enjoy!

Nutrition: calories 100, fat 5, fiber 1, carbs 1, protein 9

Chicken Meatballs

Hurry up and make these amazing meatballs today!

Preparation time: 10 minutes

Cooking time: 15 minutes

Servings: 3

Ingredients:

- 1 pound chicken meat, ground
- Salt and black pepper to the taste
- 2 tablespoons ranch dressing
- ½ cup almond flour
- ¼ cup cheddar cheese, grated
- 1 tablespoon dry ranch seasoning
- ¼ cup hot sauce+ some more for serving
- 1 egg

Directions:

1. In a bowl, mix chicken meat with salt, pepper, ranch dressing, flour, dry ranch seasoning, cheddar cheese, hot sauce and the egg and Stir very well.
2. Shape 9 meatballs, place them all on a lined baking sheet and bake at 500 degrees F for 15 minutes.

3. Serve chicken meatballs with hot sauce on the side.

Enjoy!

Nutrition: calories 156, fat 11, fiber 1, carbs 2, protein 12

Tasty Grilled Chicken Wings

You will have these done in no time and they will taste wonderful!

Preparation time: 2 hours and 10 minutes

Cooking time: 15 minutes

Servings: 5

Ingredients:

- 2 pounds wings
- Juice from 1 lime
- 1 handful cilantro, chopped
- 2 garlic cloves, minced
- 1 jalapeno pepper, chopped
- 3 tablespoons coconut oil
- Salt and black pepper to the taste
- Lime wedges for serving
- Ranch dip for serving

Directions:

1. In a bowl, mix lime juice with cilantro, garlic, jalapeno, coconut oil, salt and pepper and whisk well.
2. Add chicken wings, toss to coat and keep in the fridge for 2 hours.

3. Place chicken wings on your preheated grill over medium high heat and cook for 7 minutes on each side.

4. Serve these amazing chicken wings with ranch did and lime wedges on the side.

Enjoy!

Nutrition: calories 132, fat 5, fiber 1, carbs 4, protein 12

Easy Baked Chicken

It's a very simple keto chicken recipe!

Preparation time: 10 minutes

Cooking time: 20 minutes

Servings: 4

Ingredients:

- 4 bacon strips
- 4 chicken breasts
- 3 green onions, chopped
- 4 ounces ranch dressing
- 1 ounce coconut aminos
- 2 tablespoons coconut oil
- 4 ounces cheddar cheese, grated

Directions:

1. Heat up a pan with the oil over high heat, add chicken breasts, cook for 7 minutes, flip and cook for 7 more minutes.
2. Meanwhile, heat up another pan over medium high heat, add bacon, cook until it's crispy, transfer to paper towels, drain grease and crumble.

3. Transfer chicken breast to a baking dish, add coconut aminos, crumbled bacon, cheese and green onions on top, introduce in your oven, set on broiler and cook at a high temperature for 5 minutes more.

4. Divide between plates and serve hot.

Enjoy!

Nutrition: calories 450, fat 24, fiber 0, carbs 3, protein 60

Special Italian Chicken

This is an Italian style keto dish we really appreciate!

Preparation time: 10 minutes

Cooking time: 20 minutes

Servings: 4

Ingredients:

- ¼ cup olive oil
- 1 red onion, chopped
- 4 chicken breasts, skinless and boneless
- 4 garlic cloves, minced
- Salt and black pepper to the taste
- ½ cup Italian olives, pitted and chopped
- 4 anchovy fillets, chopped
- 1 tablespoon capers, chopped
- 1 pound tomatoes, chopped
- ½ teaspoon red chili flakes

Directions:

1. Season chicken with salt and pepper and rub with half of the oil.

2. Place into a pan which you've heated over high temperature, cook for 2 minutes, flip and cook for 2 minutes more.
3. Introduce chicken breasts in the oven at 450 degrees F and bake for 8 minutes.
4. Take chicken out of the oven and divide between plates.
5. Heat up the same pan with the rest of the oil over medium heat, add capers, onion, garlic, olives, anchovies, chili flakes and capers, stir and cook for 1 minute.
6. Add salt, pepper and tomatoes, stir and cook for 2 minutes more.
7. Drizzle this over chicken breasts and serve.

Enjoy!

Nutrition: calories 400, fat 20, fiber 1, carbs 2, protein 7

Simple Lemon Chicken

You'll soon see how easy this keto recipe is!

Preparation time: 10 minutes

Cooking time: 45 minutes

Servings: 6

Ingredients:

- 1 whole chicken, cut into medium pieces
- Salt and black pepper to the taste
- Juice from 2 lemons
- Zest from 2 lemons
- Lemon rinds from 2 lemons

Directions:

1. Put chicken pieces in a baking dish, season with salt and pepper to the taste and drizzle lemon juice.
2. Toss to coat well, add lemon zest and lemon rinds, introduce in the oven at 375 degrees F and bake for 45 minutes.
3. Discard lemon rinds, divide chicken between plates, drizzle sauce from the baking dish over it and serve.

Enjoy!

Nutrition: calories 334, fat 24, fiber 2, carbs 4.5, protein 27

Fried Chicken And Paprika Sauce

It's very healthy and it will make a great dinner idea!

Preparation time: 10 minutes

Cooking time: 20 minutes

Servings: 5

Ingredients:

- 1 tablespoon coconut oil
- 3 and ½ pounds chicken breasts
- 1 cup chicken stock
- 1 and ¼ cups yellow onion, chopped
- 1 tablespoon lime juice
- ¼ cup coconut milk
- 2 teaspoons paprika
- 1 teaspoon red pepper flakes
- 2 tablespoons green onions, chopped
- Salt and black pepper to the taste

Directions:

1. Heat up a pan with the oil over medium high heat, add chicken, cook for 2 minutes on each side, transfer to a plate and leave aside.

2. Reduce heat to medium, add onions to the pan and cook for 4 minutes.
3. Add stock, coconut milk, pepper flakes, paprika, lime juice, salt and pepper and stir well.
4. Return chicken to the pan, add more salt and pepper, cover pan and cook for 15 minutes.
5. Divide between plates and serve.

Enjoy!

Nutrition: calories 140, fat 4, fiber 3, carbs 3, protein 6

Amazing Chicken Fajitas

Are you in the mood for some tasty Mexican style food? Then, try this next idea!

Preparation time: 10 minutes

Cooking time: 15 minutes

Servings: 4

Ingredients:

- 2 pounds chicken breasts, skinless, boneless and cut into strips
- 1 teaspoon garlic powder
- 1 teaspoon chili powder
- 2 teaspoons cumin
- 2 tablespoons lime juice
- Salt and black pepper to the taste
- 1 teaspoon sweet paprika
- 2 tablespoons coconut oil
- 1 teaspoon coriander, ground
- 1 green bell pepper, sliced
- 1 red bell pepper, sliced
- 1 yellow onion, sliced

- 1 tablespoon cilantro, chopped
- 1 avocado, pitted, peeled and sliced
- 2 limes, cut into wedges

Directions:
1. In a bowl, mix lime juice with chili powder, cumin, salt, pepper, garlic powder, paprika and coriander and stir.
2. Add chicken pieces and toss to coat well.
3. Heat up a pan with half of the oil over medium high heat, add chicken, cook for 3 minutes on each side and transfer to a bowl.
4. Heat up the pan with the rest of the oil over medium heat, add onion and all bell peppers, stir and cook for 6 minutes.
5. Return chicken to pan, add more salt and pepper, stir and divide between plates.
6. Top with avocado, lime wedges and cilantro and serve.

Enjoy!

Nutrition: calories 240, fat 10, fiber 2, carbs 5, protein 20

Skillet Chicken And Mushrooms

The combination is absolutely delicious! We guarantee it!

Preparation time: 10 minutes

Cooking time: 30 minutes

Servings: 4

Ingredients:

- 4 chicken thighs
- 2 cups mushrooms, sliced
- ¼ cup ghee
- Salt and black pepper to the taste
- ½ teaspoon onion powder
- ½ teaspoon garlic powder
- ½ cup water
- 1 teaspoon Dijon mustard
- 1 tablespoon tarragon, chopped

Directions:

1. Heat up a pan with half of the ghee over medium high heat, add chicken thighs, season them with salt, pepper, garlic powder and onion powder, cook the for 3 minutes on each side and transfer to a bowl.

2. Heat up the same pan with the rest of the ghee over medium high heat, add mushrooms, stir and cook for 5 minutes.
3. Add mustard and water and stir well.
4. Return chicken pieces to the pan, stir, cover and cook for 15 minutes.
5. Add tarragon, stir, cook for 5 minutes, divide between plates and serve.

Enjoy!

Nutrition: calories 453, fat 32, fiber 6, carbs 1, protein 36

Chicken And Olives Tapenade

Everyone will be impressed with this keto dish!

Preparation time: 10 minutes

Cooking time: 10 minutes

Servings: 2

Ingredients:

- 1 chicken breast cut into 4 pieces
- 2 tablespoons coconut oil
- 3 garlic cloves, crushed
- ½ cup olives tapenade

For the tapenade:

- 1 cup black olives, pitted
- Salt and black pepper to the taste
- 2 tablespoons olive oil
- ¼ cup parsley, chopped
- 1 tablespoons lemon juice

Directions:

1. In your food processor, mix olives with salt, pepper, 2 tablespoons olive oil, lemon juice and parsley, blend very well and transfer to a bowl.

2. Heat up a pan with the coconut oil over medium heat, add garlic, stir and cook for 2 minutes.
3. Add chicken pieces and cook for 4 minutes on each side.
4. Divide chicken on plates and top with the olives tapenade.

Enjoy!

Nutrition: calories 130, fat 12, fiber 0, carbs 3, protein 20

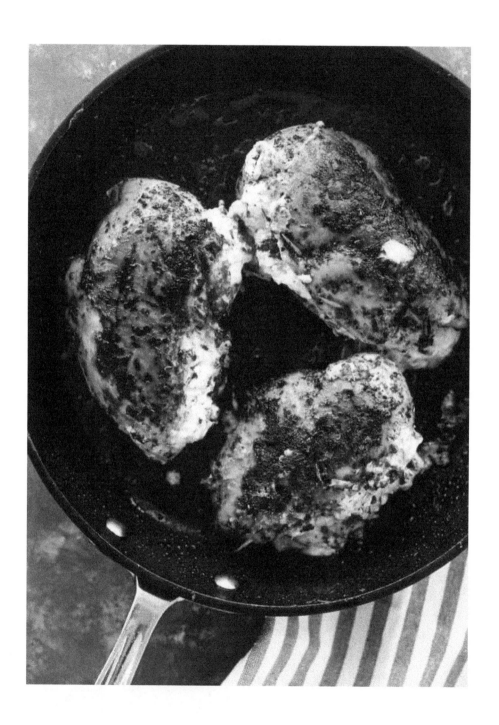

Conclusion

This is really a life changing cookbook. It shows you everything
you need to know about the Ketogenic diet and it helps you get
started.

You now know some of the best and most popular Ketogenic
recipes in the world.

We have something for everyone's taste!

So, don't hesitate too much and start your new life as a follower of
the Ketogenic diet!

Get your hands on this special recipes collection and start cooking
in this new, exciting and healthy way!

Have a lot of fun and enjoy your Ketogenic diet!